THE SCALE COMPANION

How to Find Your Ideal Body Weight

by
Ronda Gates
Frank I. Katch
Victor L. Katch

Cover Design and Illustrations by Eleni Alexandridou, International Fashion Center, Thessaloniki, Greece
Back Cover by Dave Fabik
Desktop Publishing by Crush Designs
Edited by Mary Monroe
Published by 4-Heart Press, a division of LIFESTYLES by Ronda Gates
Copyright 1998 by Ronda Gates, Frank I. Katch, and Victor L. Katch

The copyright for body composition tables in *THE SCALE COMPANION* is owned by Frank I. Katch, Victor L. Katch, William D. McArdle, and Fitness Technologies Press (1132 Lincoln Avenue, Ann Arbor, MI 48104). All rights reserved.

No part of *THE SCALE COMPANION* may be reproduced, stored in a retrieval system, or transmitted in any form or by any means: electronic, mechanical, photocopying recording or otherwise, without the prior written permission of the publisher or copyright holders.

Gates, Ronda.
    The Scale Companion : How To Find Your Ideal Body Weight / by Ronda Gates, Frank I. Katch, Victor L. Katch.
    p. cm.
    Includes bibliographical references.
    Preassigned LCCN: 97-97144
    ISBN: 1-878319-01-9

    1. Weight loss. Weight loss -- Miscellanea. 3. Body image. I. Katch, Frank I. II. Katch, Victor L. III. Title.

RM222.2.G38 1998   613.25
                                QBI97-41502

ISBN #1-878319-01-9

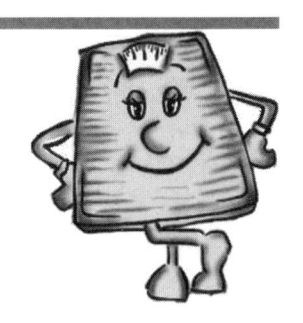

TABLE OF CONTENTS

INTRODUCTION

Why The Scale Doesn't Tell The Real Story 7
Making Friends With Your Scale (It's Just A Number!) 8
The Rest Of The Story... 9
Using *THE SCALE COMPANION* 11
A Technique You Can Trust 12

SECTION ONE—Smart Body Talk

Are You Scale-Crazy? 13
The Surprising Truth About The Scale 15
Some Guidelines Before You Get Started 17
Celebrate The Lean! 18
Why This Focus On Lean Mass? 19
How Much Body Fat Should You Have? 21
Can I Have No Body Fat? 22
The Gender Difference 23
Body Composition 101 24
Is There An Easier Way? 27
Finding Your Ideal Weight 28
The Importance Of The Lean-to-Fat Ratio 30

SECTION TWO—How To Use *THE SCALE COMPANION*

All You Need	33
Tips For Using The Tape	34
Body Sites Measured By Age And Gender	36
The Technique	37
The Tables	
Young Men	38
Older Men	40
Young Women	42
Older Women	44
One More Example Before You Start	46

SECTION THREE—Now It's Your Turn

Getting Ready	47
Step One: Gathering The Data	48
Step Two: Using The Data	51
Step Three: Calculating Your Realistic Weight Goal	52
Surprising Results!	53
A Fantasy Calculation	54

SECTION FOUR—Smart Resources

The Rest Of YOUR Story	55
Other Books Published By Authors	56
Additional Reading	57
Mailing Addresses	58
E-mail Addresses	58
Web Sites	58
Speaking Services And Program Development	58
Biographies	
Ronda Gates	59
Frank Katch	60
Victor Katch	61

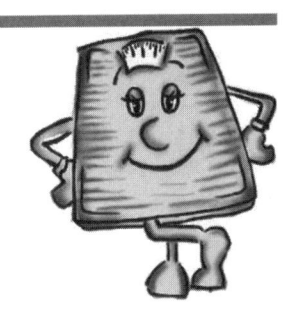

Frank Katch and Victor Katch provided the age and gender specific equations to predict body fat percentage based on girth measurements. They are based on research done in their laboratories at the University of Massachusetts and the University of Michigan.

Ronda Gates is responsible for all text. It is based on her experience in the fields of fitness and weight management.

Introduction

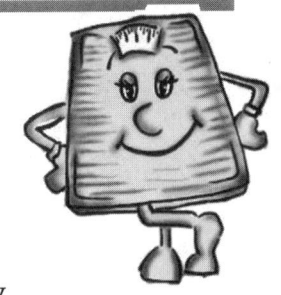

Why The Scale Doesn't Tell the Real Story

There are people who want you to think that when it comes to weight and health, the number on the scale says it all.

Don't believe them for a minute.

Unfortunately, we have been conditioned to think that this number is so important that *we often step on a scale to measure our weight but end up measuring our self worth.* This unrealistic relationship with the scale—which knows little tolerance for human individuality or diversity—haunts some of us from as far back as childhood. For others, it begins in adolescence or the first time we believe we don't "measure up" to some standard or "norm."

Once we have given so much power over our self-image to the scale, all sorts of unhealthy behaviors set in. We engage in daily weight wars with ourselves, rigidly watching every ounce and morsel. We use the number on the scale as a way to confirm all our worst fears of inadequacy and failure. Or we defiantly decide to ignore the scale—and our health along with it.

It's no wonder people have angrily started throwing away their bathroom scales! But is that really the answer?

The Scale Companion

Making Friends With Your Scale (It's Just a Number!)

We believe that it's possible to change your relationship to the scale and learn to use it as a valuable, self-empowering (not self-diminishing) tool. A healthy relationship with the scale begins with the awareness that scale weight does not define who you are, or how healthy you are. Scientists have clearly shown the scale simply does not tell the whole story. Perhaps you have read about the male flight attendant suspended by his employer because at 5' 7" and 178 pounds he was too "heavy" to meet the airline height-weight criteria. This very fit young man exercised regularly and lifted weights. His weight was evenly distributed on his obviously strong body. A body composition assessment revealed that only 7% of his total weight was fat. He knew the scale revealed only his total weight, not that most of that weight was muscle, not fat. This young man also knew that body fat goals for men range from 10% to 20% of their total weight. He might be "overweight" by airline criteria, but he was not overfat. The report of his body composition assessment empowered him to successfully challenge his employer. He sued the airline. And he won.

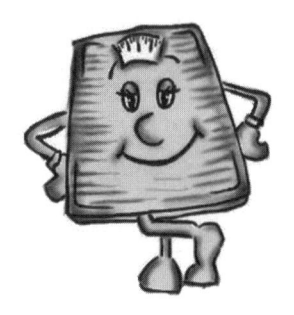

Introduction

The Rest of the Story...

THE SCALE COMPANION was developed to tell you what the scale alone cannot. It is designed to help you use the scale as one part of a self-awareness equation that emphasizes body composition, not scale weight.

Body composition refers to how much of your total body weight is fat tissue and how much is non-fat tissue. Before we go any further, let's clarify one thing: it is not our ultimate goal to find out how much body fat you have. Much like the determination of your scale weight, your body fat percentage is merely one necessary step to the discovery of a wealth of information that can help you reach optimum health. (The last thing we want to do is attach too much importance to yet another tyrannical number!) Our real objective is to determine how much lean mass, or muscle, bone and other non-fat tissue, you have. Empowered with this information, you will be able to calculate your ideal weight. Ideal weight refers to the weight that is most reasonable and healthy for your particular body .

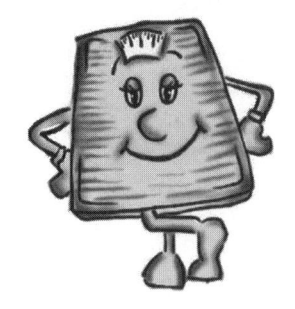

Most of the people we know who have used **THE SCALE COMPANION** have been surprised to learn that their ideal weight is actually quite different than what they initially imagined it to be. They are relieved to discover that their ideal weight is far more attainable than they thought! This is because, unlike methods that use scale weight or body fat percentage as the only criteria, **THE SCALE COMPANION** focuses on the largest, most active, most powerful part of your unique body composition-- your lean mass.

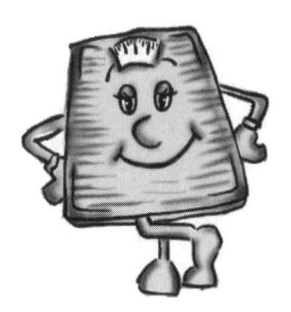

Introduction

Using *THE SCALE COMPANION*

THE SCALE COMPANION consists of this instructional booklet and the enclosed tape measure. It has been designed to give you:
- *convenient ease of use*
- *complete privacy*
- *dependable accuracy*

All you have to do is carefully take three measurements appropriate for your age and gender with the enclosed tape measure. These measurements are listed on page 36. Next, you will follow the step-by-step instructions to calculate your percentage of body fat. Then you will be guided through the process necessary to calculate your ideal weight. With this knowledge, you can develop an action plan that uses sound exercise and eating strategies to reach your goal.

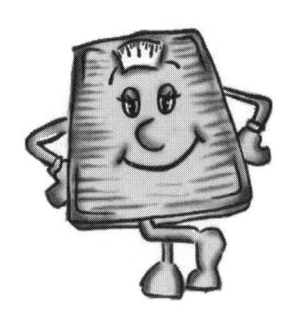

The Scale Companion

A Technique You Can Trust

You can be confident that *THE SCALE COMPANION* is a credible, dependable assessment method, recognized and accepted for some time by leaders in the field of exercise science and fitness training. The techniques described in this book were perfected in professors Frank and Victor Katch's respected research laboratories at the Universities of Massachusetts and Michigan. Each have published many scientific journals and describe their work in detail in several of their college textbooks. (See the resource list on pages 56 and 57 of this booklet.) Ronda Gates has successfully used *THE SCALE COMPANION* as a first step in her many years of work as a successful weight management coach.

For further help using this body composition method, we encourage you to:

- *consult with a health promotion professional*
- *write to us at the addresses on page 58*
- *send us E-mail (addresses listed on page 58)*
- *visit our web sites at the addresses listed on page 58 for additional education and Smart Bargains*

We hope *THE SCALE COMPANION* helps you determine and achieve an individualized, accurate, realistic weight goal.

The best of health to you,

Ronda Gates, Frank Katch, Victor Katch

Section One - Smart Body Talk

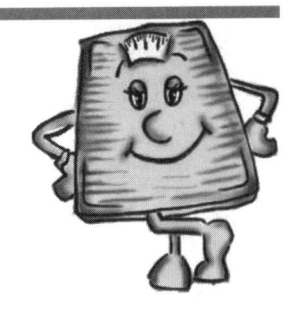

Are You Scale-Crazy?

Do you walk around asking people how much they weigh? Probably not. Chances are, however, you may be one of the millions of Americans who spend a lot of time worrying about their weight. You may even have developed the subtle but persistent habit of weighing yourself one or more times each day. If the scale's reading fits into some predetermined range, you're happy. On the other hand, when the scale reveals a number above that preferred range, you may give yourself a mental beating. "I'm such a fool." "I shouldn't have eaten that dessert!" "I should not have skipped my exercise class!"

It's easy to understand how we became so phobic about the information we get when we step on a scale. The media are constantly bombarding us with the message that happy people are skinny and beautiful. Even when we discover that the people in these ads are genetically predisposed to be thin, have over-exercised or temporarily starved themselves to acquire their lean look, or have images that are computer enhanced, we often continue to strive for an unrealistically low weight.

Physicians and insurance companies also mislead us by continuing to rely on fifty-year-old height/weight charts to predict what our "goal weight" should be. Even though they know it is impossible to make a realistic determination of health risk based solely on how much we weigh, too many health professionals continue to weigh us anyway. They compare our results to a chart, and surprise! They declare that we need to lose (or gain) weight to reach a magic number. Unfortunately, this magic number is often not the right goal for us.

This obsessive reliance disregards what scientists have learned about the relationship between body weight and our predisposition to disease.

For many of us stepping on a scale to measure our weight becomes a measurement of our self worth.

Section One

The Surprising Truth About the Scale

Scientists have learned that it is not our weight in relation to our height that is most important to our health—it is the relation of our fat to our lean mass that matters most. Research shows that people who have a higher percentage of body fat tend to have a higher risk for diseases such as high blood pressure, heart attacks, strokes, diabetes and cancer. Moreover some people who appear skinny can have a high percentage of body fat and some people (like the flight attendant in our introduction) can appear to be overweight but have a low percentage of body fat.

Think about this paradox for a moment. The terms "underweight" and "thin" and the terms "overweight" and "fat" are not necessarily synonymous. It is quite possible for an "overweight" person, especially a very fit person with lots of muscle, to have very little stored body fat. It is also possible for a "skinny" low weight person who diets a lot and doesn't exercise to have too much fat. Ronda has seen many examples of this in her years of experience doing body composition assessment throughout the United States.

How can this happen?

It's easy. Fat can be hidden inside the body in such a way that you can be overfat without seeming to be overweight at all. A sedentary person may have a low total body weight but be overfat because he has none of the muscle development that occurs with exercise. On the other hand, muscular or strong athletes often exceed weight recommendations for their sex and height, but they are not fat. A misinformed coach or physician might even encourage such an athlete to lose weight without concern for his or her proportion of lean to fat, and then wonder why the athlete is not successful at weight loss. A body that isn't overfat resists giving up healthy non-fat tissue; it has little weight to lose.

We know now that height/weight charts to determine obesity can be misleading statistical data accumulated primarily by insurance companies in the 1930's, before we knew about body composition, or the relationship between lean mass, fat and total weight.

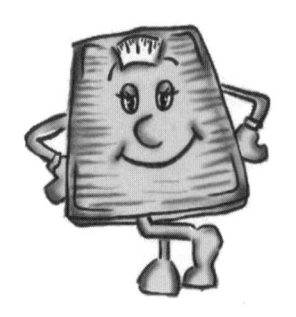

Section One

Some Guidelines Before You Get Started

Before we explain how to make THE SCALE COMPANION work for you, we'd like to suggest some guidelines to keep in mind as you undertake this process:

Don't let mere numbers determine how you feel about yourself. Remember, your body weight and body fat percentage are simply self-awareness tools. Don't give these numbers more power than they deserve! Try to avoid negative judgments and self-talk.

Don't run the risk of getting frustrated before you give yourself enough time to make permanent, lasting change. Continually remind yourself that the goal of this process is to improve your health over time, not to make miraculous changes overnight.

Keep your sense of humor and don't take yourself too seriously! There is tremendous physical diversity in the human population, and very few people (including models and celebrities) are completely satisfied with their physical appearance. We weren't meant to have identical shapes and sizes, and we weren't meant to fit an idealized version of "perfect".

Now, let's take a closer look at what you should know about lean mass and body fat percentage.

Celebrating the Lean!

It's tempting to focus strictly on our body fat percentage and ignore the part of us that isn't fat! A more affirming approach is to recognize and celebrate our lean selves.

When you exclude body fat, the remainder of your weight is described by scientists as "fat-free weight." Fat-free weight includes muscle, bone, water, connective tissues, organs, skin, hair, teeth—everything except essential and stored body fat. We also use the term "lean mass" to describe fat-free weight. Technically, lean mass or lean weight includes a small amount of essential fat. Health and fitness professionals take even greater liberty with these terms. When they encourage us to maintain, build or gain "lean mass," they are actually talking about muscle mass. In **THE SCALE COMPANION** we will also use "lean mass" to describe muscle mass.

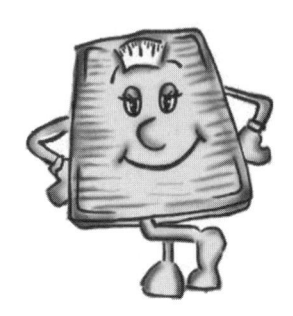

Section One

Why This Focus On Lean Mass?

Your lean mass, or muscle, is the most active component of your body weight. Your lean mass uses calories for every function of your body, including all the muscle work you do on a minute-to-minute basis. Generally speaking, whether you are sitting around or running around, the more muscle you have, the more calories you are likely to burn. You get this additional muscle power with exercise and strength training.

No matter what you hear or read, only exercise can make you burn more calories with the muscle you have.

Suppose two friends, both 5' 5" and 150 pounds, take a two-mile walk together. Barbara is an active exerciser. In a body composition assessment she learned that her lean mass comprises 75% or 112.5 pounds of her total weight. Barbara's friend Marie is sedentary. Only 65% or 97.5 pounds of Marie's weight is lean mass. Barbara has 15 more pounds of lean mass than Marie. Most of Barbara's extra weight is muscle. On their two-mile walk, Barbara burns more calories than Marie.

If they continued to walk daily, Barbara is also likely to burn more stored body fat than Marie. And if Barbara's calorie intake did not increase she would also lose more fat weight.

Suppose both of these women decide they would like to run in a local race. Both want to lose weight because it is likely to help them run more comfortably and efficiently. They want to lose fat weight, not lean mass weight, because lean mass is the engine that powers their muscles. The only way these women could accurately determine an ideal weight is with a body composition assessment.

Where does lean mass fit into this calculation for a goal weight? If you know how much lean mass you have and if you have a goal for body composition, you can quickly make the calculations necessary to predict your ideal weight. With that goal in mind, a smart exercise and smart eating program that supports weight loss of about two pounds a week can virtually assure that your weight lost will be fat only. Weight loss programs that promise more than two pounds of weight loss per week will generate a loss of some fat and water along with fat-free mass (including the muscle that burns stored fat).

We encourage fat loss, rather than just weight loss. That's why we use lean mass to compute ideal weight. *THE SCALE COMPANION* is based on maintaining your current lean mass and decreasing your percentage of body fat to a healthy level.

It doesn't make sense to set a goal weight until you know your lean mass and body fat percentage.

Section One

What Should Your Body Fat Percentage Be?

That's a good question. If you were to ask five experts, "What is the 'ideal' range for body fat?" you might get five different answers. However, most would agree that a healthy (ideal) range for most women falls between 20% and 30% of total body weight. For men, the range is from 10% to 20% of total body weight.

IDEAL BODY FAT PERCENTAGE
Women: 20-30% of body weight
Men: 10-20% of body weight

Can I Have *No* Body Fat?

It's impossible, even in severe starvation, to have no body fat. Your body cannot function without some fat. This minimal amount described as "essential fat" occurs in bone marrow, as part of the internal organs (heart, intestines, kidneys, for example) and in the central nervous system (the brain and spinal cord).

About 3% of a man's total body fat consists of essential fat. Women require more body fat than men for childbearing and other hormone-related functions. About 12% of their total body fat is essential fat. Women and men who exercise too much or starve themselves can drop below this minimum amount. This can have serious health impairing consequences.

**CAVEAT: If you are a woman old enough to menstruate, your body's internal system warns you when body fat levels get too low. You stop menstruating.
Seek medical advice if this happens to you.**

THE GENDER DIFFERENCE

If A Man Has About 3% And A Woman About 12% Essential Fat, Why Are The Ideal Percentages Higher?

In addition to essential fat, your body has "stored fat." Approximately one-half of this stored fat is located just beneath the skin surface. It is called subcutaneous fat (sub = beneath; cutaneous = skin). Most of the remainder of your stored fat surrounds your internal organs or is between the layers of your muscles.

For men and women, stored fat exceeds the amount of essential fat. Close to 13% of a woman's total weight is stored fat. For a man, stored fat occupies about 12% of total weight. Although men and women have almost equal amounts of stored fat, the significant difference in essential fat results in different total body fat percentages. Add the essential and stored fat for men, and the total fat content averages 15% (3% essential fat plus 12% stored fat). Women average 25% fat (12% essential + 13% storage).

Allowing for genetic variability among individuals, and differences in bone density among ethnic groups, it's easy to understand why the average range for men is 10-20% and for women 20-30% of total weight.

Remember, it does not matter what that total weight is.

	Men	**Women**
Essential	3%	12%
Stored Fat	+12%	+13%
Total (average)	15%	25%

Body Composition 101

There are two basic procedures for determining body composition. The first measures body composition directly on human cadavers. For obvious reasons, this is not a popular method, but it does provide scientists with useful facts about the fat, muscle, and bone content of humans. This information is used to develop measurement methods that health and fitness professionals use to calculate the body composition of living people. These methods include hydrostatic weighing, skinfolds, electronic instrumentation, and girth or circumferential measurements.

Let's look briefly at these methods.

HYDROSTATIC WEIGHING

The gold standard for body composition assessment is called hydrostatic weighing or underwater weighing. Sometimes it is described as "getting dunked." To be assessed in this way, you sit in a chair surrounded by water. The chair is suspended from a scale similar to the one you might see at a produce store. When you are ready to begin the assessment, you exhale fully, then lower your head under the water and remain as still as possible for about five seconds. In that brief time the technician reads your underwater weight on the scale. That measurement is entered into a mathematical equations which compute the body fat percentage of your total weight.

If you have a lot of bone and muscle (which is more dense than fat) you will weigh more under the water. If you have a lot of stored body fat you will not weigh as much. In terms of this underwater weighing method, it is a compliment if someone says, "You're dense!"

Since your ability to float is also affected by age, lung volume, and water temperature, underwater weighing is a complex procedure. It is usually reserved for exercise physiology laboratories in universities, government physiology centers, sports medicine facilities, and some health and athletic clubs.

SKINFOLDS

The skinfold or "pinch" test is another common method for assessing body composition. This inexpensive, easy technique gives values for body fat similar to the underwater weighing procedures. In skinfold assessment, a special caliper measures the thickness of skin plus subcutaneous fat at several sites on your body (typically back of upper arm, upper back, abdomen, hips, mid-thigh). The values for skinfolds are then entered into an age- and sex-specific equation that estimates body fat percentage. Skinfold assessment can be accurate in the hands of an experienced assessor. However, with insufficient practice, or if two different assessors take measurements at the same sites (days, weeks or months apart), "pinched" values for body fat can be in error by 100% or more! There are electronic calipers that calibrate the pinch of the tool and make the necessary calculations via a computer chip in the caliper. Electronic skinfold calipers make skinfold assessment easy for professionals who do a lot of body composition assessment.

ELECTRONIC INSTRUMENTATION

Some manufacturers claim their sophisticated equipment can accurately measure your body's fat content, based on the resistance (or impedance) of a low voltage electric charge passed through an electrode on your finger to an electrode on your foot. Another electronic method uses an infrared sensor to measure the thickness of subcutaneous fat on your upper arm.

Both of these methods for assessing body composition are speedy and require little training. Because there are so many variables that need to be controlled to give accurate and repeatable results most body composition experts discourage their use. Imagine the frustration of getting assessed using one of these methods, beginning an exercise program, eating sensibly, then 3 months later having a repeat assessment that reports your body fat has not decreased. Although the technician may tell you this is because your hydration level is different from the previous assessment it does little to support a client's enthusiasm for maintaining their program.

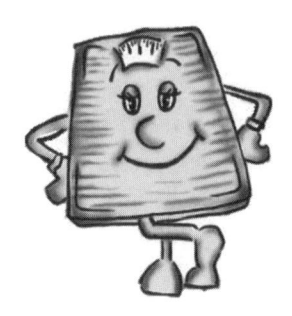

Section One

Is There An Easier Way?

Yes! *THE SCALE COMPANION* is much easier. You use a tape to measure yourself at specific sites for your age and gender. After you record these "girth" measurements, you turn to page 38 and consult the appropriate chart to translate your measurements into research based "constants". Then, after making some simple calculations, your body fat percentage is revealed. After a few simple calculations you'll know your ideal weight.

With **THE SCALE COMPANION**—the tape measure, charts and this booklet—you have everything you need to proceed through this step-by-step process to assess your body composition and determine your ideal weight. This non-invasive assessment can be repeated in private and at your convenience. Best of all, unlike some procedures, girth measurements can be mastered quickly. Because you are measuring various sites on your body, girth measurements also give you a better understanding of where you "carry" extra fat.

The charts that you will use to compute your percent body fat are based on the scientific studies of exercise physiologists Frank and Victor Katch. These charts are used in college textbooks and have been published in the *American Journal of Clinical Nutrition* and *Human Biology*. The studies by the Drs. Katch demonstrate that the accuracy of girth measurements is 3.5% or less when compared to the more complicated hydrostatic method described previously.

Finding Your Ideal Weight

Let's look again at Marie, our 5' 5", 150-pound overfat friend who takes those two-mile walks with Barbara. Marie's actual weight is 150 pounds. She wants to lose 25 pounds and weigh 125 pounds. She chose that number because she read a magazine article that suggested a woman should start with a base weight of 100 pounds and add 5 pounds for every inch of height over five feet.

However, when Marie took her girth measurements she discovered she had 35% body fat or 52.5 pounds of fat and 97.5 pounds of lean mass. If Marie sets her new goal weight to include a body fat percentage goal of 25%, she's simultaneously setting a goal for her lean mass to be 75% of her total weight (100% actual weight – 25% fat weight = 75% lean mass weight). Remember, Marie wants to lose fat weight, not lean mass because that is the valuable part of her body that includes her calorie-burning muscle.

When we divide Marie's goal of 75% lean mass into her current 97.5 pounds of lean, we discover what her weight will be when she reaches her goal of 25% body fat. (This assumes she doesn't go on any crazy diet, but instead attempts to reduce her fat weight with a sensible exercise and nutrition plan.) Here is the calculation:

97.5 pounds of lean mass ÷ 0.75 = 130 pounds.

Marie's goal weight is 130 pounds. If we subtract that goal weight from her current weight of 150 pounds, she has only 20 pounds to lose, not 25. If Marie adds strength training to her exercise program, chances are she will increase her lean mass at the same time that she loses fat weight. If she works hard and gains five pounds of lean mass, her new lean mass will be 102.5 pounds. Her goal weight at 25% fat will now be 136.6:

102.5 pounds of lean mass ÷ .75 = 136.6 pounds.

Marie has also increased her lean-to-fat ratio.

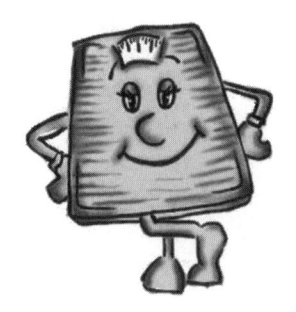

The Importance Of The Lean-to-Fat Ratio

The lean-to-fat ratio is a relative value to help you understand the beauty of having more muscle and less fat. Your lean-to-fat ratio is computed by dividing the weight of your lean mass by your pounds of fat.

Knowing your lean-to-fat ratio gives you another useful parameter to begin, continue, or improve your fitness program. Sedentary Marie provides us with a good example. With 97.5 pounds of fat-free mass and 52.5 pounds of fat, her lean-to-fat ratio is 1.8 (97.5 ÷ 52.5 = 1.8). We would say she has a low lean-to-fat ratio (too much fat and lower than normal muscle mass).

If Marie adopts a smart exercise and smart eating program, we predict her goal weight will be 130 pounds. She'd still have 97.5 pounds of lean mass but her fat weight will be down to 32.5 pounds. Marie's lean-to-fat ratio will now be 3.0 (97.5 ÷ 32.5 = 3.0).

This is a significant change. We would cheer Marie's increase in her lean-to-fat ratio!

Although there is no perfect or recommended ratio of lean-to-fat, the number can be particularly useful if you are committed to becoming fit. It can also help you understand that *the body can change significantly without a decrease in actual weight.*

A scale cannot reflect the higher body density that comes with a fitness program when you increase lean mass and decrease fat mass.

Section One

Here's another example. Marie's fit friend, Barbara, decides to train for a marathon. It is nine months away. In addition to logging miles to prepare for the race, Barbara trains with weights twice a week at her health club. At home she occasionally uses large rubber bands for additional resistance training. Months later Barbara knows she is fitter because her speed has improved and her clothes are loose. The loose clothes are a surprise because she hasn't lost a pound. She gets out her tape and repeats her measurements. Happily, after completing her calculation she discovers her body fat has decreased from 25 to 20% fat. She has gained as many pounds of muscle weight as she has lost in fat weight! Barbara's total weight of 150 pounds is now comprised of 120 pounds of lean mass and 30 pounds of fat. Her lean-to-fat ratio has increased from 3.0 (112.5 ÷ 37.5 = 3.0) to 4.0 (120 ÷ 30 = 4.0), Barbara has made significant changes in her body (and probably her health) without seeing the numbers on the scale move one pound!

Body composition assessment is remarkable in many ways. With **THE SCALE COMPANION**, you, too, can learn your:

- *body fat percentage*
- *pounds of fat*
- *pounds of fat-free (lean) mass*
- *ideal goal weight*
- *lean-to-fat ratio.*

Let's get started!

Section Two - How to Use
THE SCALE COMPANION

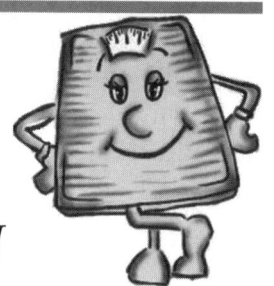

All You Need

The following pages provide:

- *instructions for using the tape measure*
- *the conversion charts necessary to convert your tape measurements to a "constant"*
- *the calculations to determine your body fat percentage*
- *instructions to determine your lean-to-fat ratio and your ideal weight.*

Don't be daunted! It's not complicated.

THE SCALE COMPANION will guide you through each step .

Tips For Using The Tape

The plastic tape measure that came with this book should last for years. Here are guidelines for effectively using the tape measure:

- Although you can report your measurements in inches, you will obtain the most accurate results if you use the side of the tape marked in centimeters (cm.).

- Don't try to keep these measurements in your head. It's much easier if you *write down* your results as you go.

- When you circle a site with the measuring tape, do it lightly. The tape should be taught but not tight. This avoids skin compression that produces lower than normal scores. *Take two measurements at each site* and use the average.

Section Two

Girth measurements are accurate for predicting body fat percentage because the three measurements needed to determine your body fat percentage are taken at sites that are specific to your age and gender. There are four categories:

- young men, ages 18 to 26
- young women, ages 18 to 26
- older men, ages 27 to 50
- older women, ages 27 to 50

After you've finished recording your girth measurements, refer to the specific chart that matches your age and gender category. Write down the constant for each of your measurements. Simple calculations will reveal your percentage of body fat.

The girth measurement strategy is most accurate for people up to age fifty (that's the limit of our research to date with the girth technique).

36 The Scale Companion

Body Sites Measured by Age and Gender

Age (Yrs)	Gender	Site Measured A	B	C
18-26	Male	Right upper arm	Abdomen	Right forearm
	Female	Abdomen	Right thigh	Right forearm
27-50	Male	Buttocks	Abdomen	Right forearm
	Female	Abdomen	Right thigh	Right calf

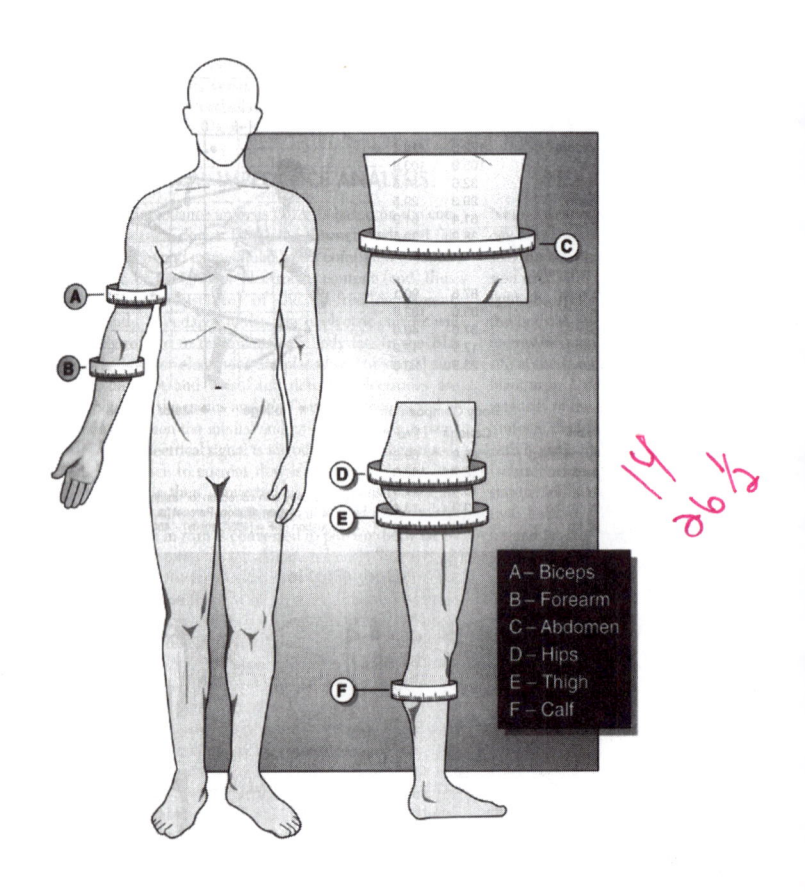

A – Biceps
B – Forearm
C – Abdomen
D – Hips
E – Thigh
F – Calf

The Technique:

Body landmarks for assessments:

1. Abdomen: one inch above the umbilicus, heels together. If a friend takes the measurement, look straight ahead, not down. Take the measurement at the end of a normal exhalation.

2. Buttocks: maximum girth with your heels together.

3. Right thigh: upper thigh just below the buttocks, feet shoulder width apart, legs straight.

4. Right upper arm: arm straight, palm up and extended in front of the body. Measure at the midpoint between the shoulder and the elbow.

5. Right forearm: maximum girth with the arm extended in front of the body with palm up.

6. Right calf: widest girth midway between the ankle and knee.

After taking the appropriate measurements for your age and sex, substitute the corresponding constants A, B, and C, into the formula listed at the bottom of your age and sex table.

NOTE: Take all measurements on the right side of the body.

Conversion Constants to Predict Body Fat for YOUNG MEN

\multicolumn{3}{c	}{Upper Arm}	\multicolumn{3}{c	}{Abdomen}	\multicolumn{3}{c}{Forearm}
in	cm	Constant A	in	cm	Constant B	in	cm	Constant C
7.00	17.78	25.91	21.00	53.34	27.56	7.00	17.78	38.01
7.25	18.41	26.83	21.25	53.97	27.88	7.25	18.41	39.37
7.50	19.05	27.76	21.50	54.61	28.21	7.50	19.05	40.72
7.75	19.68	28.68	21.75	55.24	28.54	7.75	19.68	42.08
8.00	20.32	29.61	22.00	55.88	28.87	8.00	20.32	43.44
8.25	20.95	30.53	22.25	56.51	29.20	8.25	20.95	44.80
8.50	21.59	31.46	22.50	57.15	29.52	8.50	21.59	46.15
8.75	22.22	32.38	22.75	57.78	29.85	8.75	22.22	47.51
9.00	22.86	33.31	23.00	58.42	30.18	9.00	22.86	48.87
9.25	23.49	34.24	23.25	59.05	30.51	9.25	23.49	50.23
9.50	24.13	35.16	23.50	59.69	30.84	9.50	24.13	51.58
9.75	24.76	36.09	23.75	60.32	31.16	9.75	24.76	52.94
10.00	25.40	37.01	24.00	60.96	31.49	10.00	25.40	54.30
10.25	26.03	37.94	24.25	61.59	31.82	10.25	26.03	55.65
10.50	26.67	38.86	24.50	62.23	32.15	10.50	26.67	57.01
10.75	27.30	39.79	24.75	62.86	32.48	10.75	27.30	58.37
11.00	27.94	40.71	25.00	63.50	32.80	11.00	27.94	59.73
11.25	28.57	41.64	25.25	64.13	33.13	11.25	28.57	61.08
11.50	29.21	42.56	25.50	64.77	33.46	11.50	29.21	62.44
11.75	29.84	43.49	25.75	65.40	33.79	11.75	29.84	63.80
12.00	30.48	44.41	26.00	66.04	34.12	12.00	30.48	65.16
12.25	31.11	45.34	26.25	66.67	34.44	12.25	31.11	66.51
12.50	31.75	46.26	26.50	67.31	34.77	12.50	31.75	67.87
12.75	32.38	47.19	26.75	67.94	35.10	12.75	32.38	69.23
13.00	33.02	48.11	27.00	68.58	35.43	13.00	33.02	70.59
13.25	33.65	49.04	27.25	69.21	35.76	13.25	33.65	71.94
13.50	34.29	49.96	27.50	69.85	36.09	13.50	34.29	73.30
13.75	34.92	50.89	27.75	70.48	36.41	13.75	34.92	74.66
14.00	35.56	51.82	28.00	71.12	36.74	14.00	35.56	76.02
14.25	36.19	52.74	28.25	71.75	37.07	14.25	36.19	77.37
14.50	36.83	53.67	28.50	72.39	37.40	14.50	36.83	78.73
14.75	37.46	54.59	28.75	73.02	37.73	14.75	37.46	80.09
15.00	38.10	55.52	29.00	73.66	38.05	15.00	38.10	81.45
15.25	38.73	56.44	29.25	74.29	38.38	15.25	38.73	82.80
15.50	39.37	57.37	29.50	74.93	38.71	15.50	39.37	84.16
15.75	40.00	58.29	29.75	75.56	39.04	15.75	40.00	85.52
16.00	40.64	59.22	30.00	76.20	39.37	16.00	40.64	86.88
16.25	41.27	60.14	30.25	76.83	39.69	16.25	41.27	88.23
16.50	41.91	61.07	30.50	77.47	40.02	16.50	41.91	89.59
16.75	42.54	61.99	30.75	78.10	40.35	16.75	42.54	90.95
17.00	43.18	62.92	31.00	78.74	40.68	17.00	43.18	92.31
17.25	43.81	63.84	31.25	79.37	41.01	17.25	43.81	93.66
17.50	44.45	64.77	31.50	80.01	41.33	17.50	44.45	95.02
17.75	45.08	65.69	31.75	80.64	41.66	17.75	45.08	96.38
18.00	45.72	66.62	32.00	81.28	41.99	18.00	45.72	97.74
18.25	46.35	67.54	32.25	81.91	42.32	18.25	46.35	99.09
18.50	46.99	68.47	32.50	82.55	42.65	18.50	46.99	100.45
18.75	47.62	69.40	32.75	83.18	42.97	18.75	47.62	101.81
19.00	48.26	70.32	33.00	83.82	43.30	19.00	48.26	103.17
19.25	48.89	71.25	33.25	84.45	43.63	19.25	48.89	104.52
19.50	49.53	72.17	33.50	85.09	43.96	19.50	49.53	105.88
19.75	50.16	73.10	33.75	85.72	44.29	19.75	50.16	107.24

Conversion Constants to Predict Body Fat for YOUNG MEN (cont'd.)

\multicolumn{3}{c	}{Upper Arm}	\multicolumn{3}{c	}{Abdomen}	\multicolumn{3}{c}{Forearm}
in	cm	Constant A	in	cm	Constant B	in	cm	Constant C
20.00	50.80	74.02	34.00	86.36	44.61	20.00	50.80	108.60
20.25	51.43	74.95	34.25	86.99	44.94	20.25	51.43	109.95
20.50	52.07	75.87	34.50	87.63	45.27	20.50	52.07	111.31
20.75	52.70	76.80	34.75	88.26	45.60	20.75	52.70	112.67
21.00	53.34	77.72	35.00	88.90	45.93	21.00	53.34	114.02
21.25	53.97	78.65	35.25	89.53	46.25	21.25	53.97	115.38
21.50	54.61	79.57	35.50	90.17	46.58	21.50	54.61	116.74
21.75	55.24	80.50	35.75	90.80	46.91	21.75	55.24	118.10
22.00	55.88	81.42	36.00	91.44	47.24	22.00	55.88	119.45
			36.25	92.07	47.57			
			36.50	92.71	47.89			
			36.75	93.34	48.22			
			37.00	93.98	48.55			
			37.25	94.61	48.88			
			37.50	95.25	49.21			
			37.75	95.88	49.54			
			38.00	96.52	49.86			
			38.25	97.15	50.19			
			38.50	97.79	50.52			
			38.75	98.42	50.85			
			39.00	99.06	51.18			
			39.25	99.69	51.50			
			39.50	100.33	51.83			
			39.75	100.96	52.16			
			40.00	101.60	52.49			
			40.25	102.23	52.82			
			40.50	102.87	53.14			
			40.75	103.50	53.47			
			41.00	104.14	53.80			
			41.25	104.77	54.13			
			41.50	105.41	54.46			
			41.75	106.04	54.78			
			42.00	106.68	55.11			

Young Men: Percent fat = Constant A + Constant B − Constant C − 10.2

Conversion Constants to Predict Body Fat for OLDER MEN

| \multicolumn{3}{c|}{Buttocks} | \multicolumn{3}{c|}{Abdomen} | \multicolumn{3}{c}{Forearm} |

Buttocks in	Buttocks cm	Constant A	Abdomen in	Abdomen cm	Constant B	Forearm in	Forearm cm	Constant C
28.00	71.12	29.34	25.50	64.77	22.84	7.00	17.78	21.01
28.25	71.75	29.60	25.75	65.40	23.06	7.25	18.41	21.76
28.50	72.39	29.87	26.00	66.04	23.29	7.50	19.05	22.52
28.75	73.02	30.13	26.25	66.67	23.51	7.75	19.68	23.26
29.00	73.66	30.39	26.50	67.31	23.73	8.00	20.32	24.02
29.25	74.29	30.65	26.75	67.94	23.96	8.25	20.95	24.76
29.50	74.93	30.92	27.00	68.58	24.18	8.50	21.59	25.52
29.75	75.56	31.18	27.25	69.21	24.40	8.75	22.22	26.26
30.00	76.20	31.44	27.50	69.85	24.63	9.00	22.86	27.02
30.25	76.83	31.70	27.75	70.48	24.85	9.25	23.49	27.76
30.50	77.47	31.96	28.00	71.12	25.08	9.50	24.13	28.52
30.75	78.10	32.22	28.25	71.75	25.29	9.75	24.76	29.26
31.00	78.74	32.49	28.50	72.39	25.52	10.00	25.40	30.02
31.25	79.37	32.75	28.75	73.02	25.75	10.25	26.03	30.76
31.50	80.01	33.01	29.00	73.66	25.97	10.50	26.67	31.52
31.75	80.64	33.27	29.25	74.29	26.19	10.75	27.30	32.27
32.00	81.28	33.54	29.50	74.93	26.42	11.00	27.94	33.02
32.25	81.91	33.80	29.75	75.56	26.64	11.25	28.57	33.77
32.50	82.55	34.06	30.00	76.20	26.87	11.50	29.21	34.52
32.75	83.18	34.32	30.25	76.83	27.09	11.75	29.84	35.27
33.00	83.82	34.58	30.50	77.47	27.32	12.00	30.48	36.02
33.25	84.45	34.84	30.75	78.10	27.54	12.25	31.11	36.77
33.50	85.09	35.11	31.00	78.74	27.76	12.50	31.75	37.53
33.75	85.72	35.37	31.25	79.37	27.98	12.75	32.38	38.27
34.00	86.36	35.63	31.50	80.01	28.21	13.00	33.02	39.03
34.25	86.99	35.89	31.75	80.64	28.43	13.25	33.65	39.77
34.50	87.63	36.16	32.00	81.28	28.66	13.50	34.29	40.53
34.75	88.26	36.42	32.25	81.91	28.88	13.75	34.92	41.27
35.00	88.90	36.68	32.50	82.55	29.11	14.00	35.56	42.03
35.25	89.53	36.94	32.75	83.18	29.33	14.25	36.19	42.77
35.50	90.17	37.20	33.00	83.82	29.55	14.50	36.83	43.53
35.75	90.80	37.46	33.25	84.45	29.78	14.75	37.46	44.27
36.00	91.44	37.73	33.50	85.09	30.00	15.00	38.10	45.03
36.25	92.07	37.99	33.75	85.72	30.22	15.25	38.73	45.77
36.50	92.71	38.25	34.00	86.36	30.45	15.50	39.37	46.53
36.75	93.34	38.51	34.25	86.99	30.67	15.75	40.00	47.28
37.00	93.98	38.78	34.50	87.63	30.89	16.00	40.64	48.03
37.25	94.61	39.04	34.75	88.26	31.12	16.25	41.27	48.78
37.50	95.25	39.30	35.00	88.90	31.35	16.50	41.91	49.53
37.75	95.88	39.56	35.25	89.53	31.57	16.75	42.54	50.28
38.00	96.52	39.82	35.50	90.17	31.79	17.00	43.18	51.03
38.25	97.15	40.08	35.75	90.80	32.02	17.25	43.81	51.78
38.50	97.79	40.35	36.00	91.44	32.24	17.50	44.45	52.54
38.75	98.42	40.61	36.25	92.07	32.46	17.75	45.08	53.28
39.00	99.06	40.87	36.50	92.71	32.69	18.00	45.72	54.04
39.25	99.69	41.13	36.75	93.34	32.91	18.25	46.35	54.78
39.50	100.33	41.39	37.00	93.98	33.14			
39.75	100.96	41.66	37.25	94.61	33.36			
40.00	101.60	41.92	37.50	95.25	33.58			
40.25	102.23	42.18	37.75	95.88	33.81			
40.50	102.87	42.44	38.00	96.52	34.03			
40.75	103.50	42.70	38.25	97.15	34.26			

Section Two

Conversion Constants to Predict Body Fat for OLDER MEN (cont'd.)

Buttocks			Abdomen			Forearm		
in	cm	Constant A	in	cm	Constant B	in	cm	Constant C
41.00	104.14	42.97	38.50	97.79	34.48			
41.25	104.77	43.23	38.75	98.42	34.70			
41.50	105.41	43.49	39.00	99.06	34.93			
41.75	106.04	43.75	39.25	99.69	35.15			
42.00	106.68	44.02	39.50	100.33	35.38			
42.25	107.31	44.28	39.75	100.96	35.59			
42.50	107.95	44.54	40.00	101.60	35.82			
42.75	108.58	44.80	40.25	102.23	36.05			
43.00	109.22	45.06	40.50	102.87	36.27			
43.25	109.85	45.32	40.75	103.50	36.49			
43.50	110.49	45.59	41.00	104.14	36.72			
43.75	111.12	45.85	41.25	104.77	36.94			
44.00	111.76	46.12	41.50	105.41	37.17			
44.25	112.39	46.37	41.75	106.04	37.39			
44.50	113.03	46.64	42.00	106.68	37.62			
44.75	113.66	46.89	42.25	107.31	37.87			
45.00	114.30	47.16	42.50	107.95	38.06			
45.25	114.93	47.42	42.75	108.58	38.28			
45.50	115.57	47.68	43.00	109.22	38.51			
45.75	116.20	47.94	43.25	109.85	38.73			
46.00	116.84	48.21	43.50	110.49	38.96			
46.25	117.47	48.47	43.75	111.12	39.18			
46.50	118.11	48.73	44.00	111.76	39.41			
46.75	118.74	48.99	44.25	112.39	39.63			
47.00	119.38	49.26	44.50	113.03	39.85			
47.25	120.01	49.52	44.75	113.66	40.08			
47.50	120.65	49.78	45.00	114.30	40.30			
47.75	121.28	50.04						
48.00	121.92	50.30						
48.25	122.55	50.56						
48.50	123.19	50.83						
48.75	123.82	51.09						
49.00	124.46	51.35						

Older Men: Percent fat = Constant A + Constant B - Constant C - 15.0

Table 2-3

Conversion Constants to Predict Body Fat for YOUNG WOMEN

\multicolumn{3}{c	}{Abdomen}	\multicolumn{3}{c	}{Thigh}	\multicolumn{3}{c}{Forearm}
in	cm	Constant A	in	cm	Constant B	in	cm	Constant C
20.00	50.80	26.74	14.00	35.56	29.13	6.00	15.24	25.86
20.25	51.43	27.07	14.25	36.19	29.65	6.25	15.87	26.94
20.50	52.07	27.41	14.50	36.83	30.17	6.50	16.51	28.02
20.75	52.70	27.74	14.75	37.46	30.69	6.75	17.14	29.10
21.00	53.34	28.07	15.00	38.10	31.21	7.00	17.78	30.17
21.25	53.97	28.41	15.25	38.73	31.73	7.25	18.41	31.25
21.50	54.61	28.74	15.50	39.37	32.25	7.50	19.05	32.33
21.75	55.24	29.08	15.75	40.00	32.77	7.75	19.68	33.41
22.00	55.88	29.41	16.00	40.64	33.29	8.00	20.32	34.48
22.25	56.51	29.74	16.25	41.27	33.81	8.25	20.95	35.56
22.50	57.15	30.08	16.50	41.91	34.33	8.50	21.59	36.64
22.75	57.78	30.41	16.75	42.54	34.85	8.75	22.22	37.72
23.00	58.42	30.75	17.00	43.18	35.37	9.00	22.86	38.79
23.25	59.05	31.08	17.25	43.81	35.89	9.25	23.49	39.87
23.50	59.69	31.42	17.50	44.45	36.41	9.50	24.13	40.95
23.75	60.32	31.75	17.75	45.08	36.93	9.75	24.76	42.03
24.00	60.96	32.08	18.00	45.72	37.45	10.00	25.40	43.10
24.25	61.59	32.42	18.25	46.35	37.97	10.25	26.03	44.18
24.50	62.23	32.75	18.50	46.99	38.49	10.50	26.67	45.26
24.75	62.86	33.09	18.75	47.62	39.01	10.75	27.30	46.34
25.00	63.50	33.42	19.00	48.26	39.53	11.00	27.94	47.41
25.25	64.13	33.76	19.25	48.89	40.05	11.25	28.57	48.49
25.50	64.77	34.09	19.50	49.53	40.57	11.50	29.21	49.57
25.75	65.40	34.42	19.75	50.16	41.09	11.75	29.84	50.65
26.00	66.04	34.76	20.00	50.80	41.61	12.00	30.48	51.73
26.25	66.67	35.09	20.25	51.43	42.13	12.25	31.11	52.80
26.50	67.31	35.43	20.50	52.07	42.65	12.50	31.75	53.88
26.75	67.94	35.76	20.75	52.70	43.17	12.75	32.38	54.96
27.00	68.58	36.10	21.00	53.34	43.69	13.00	33.02	56.04
27.25	69.21	36.43	21.25	53.97	44.21	13.25	33.65	57.11
27.50	69.85	36.76	21.50	54.61	44.73	13.50	34.29	58.19
27.75	70.48	37.10	21.75	55.24	45.25	13.75	34.92	59.27
28.00	71.12	37.43	22.00	55.88	45.77	14.00	35.56	60.35
28.25	71.75	37.77	22.25	56.51	46.29	14.25	36.19	61.42
28.50	72.39	38.10	22.50	57.15	46.81	14.50	36.83	62.50
28.75	73.02	38.43	22.75	57.78	47.33	14.75	37.46	63.58
29.00	73.66	38.77	23.00	58.42	47.85	15.00	38.10	64.66
29.25	74.29	39.10	23.25	59.05	48.37	15.25	38.73	65.73
29.50	74.93	39.44	23.50	59.69	48.89	15.50	39.37	66.81
29.75	75.56	39.77	23.75	60.32	49.41	15.75	40.00	67.89
30.00	76.20	40.11	24.00	60.96	49.93	16.00	40.64	68.97
30.25	76.83	40.44	24.25	61.59	50.45	16.25	41.27	70.04
30.50	77.47	40.77	24.50	62.23	50.97	16.50	41.91	71.12
30.75	78.10	41.11	24.75	62.86	51.49	16.75	42.54	72.20
31.00	78.74	41.44	25.00	63.50	52.01	17.00	43.18	73.28
31.25	79.37	41.78	25.25	64.13	52.53	17.25	43.81	74.36
31.50	80.01	42.11	25.50	64.77	53.05	17.50	44.45	75.43
31.75	80.64	42.45	25.75	65.40	53.57	17.75	45.08	76.51
32.00	81.28	42.78	26.00	66.04	54.09	18.00	45.72	77.59
32.25	81.91	43.11	26.25	66.67	54.61	18.25	46.35	78.67
32.50	82.55	43.45	26.50	67.31	55.13	18.50	46.99	79.74
32.75	83.18	43.78	26.75	67.94	55.65	18.75	47.62	80.82

Section Two

Conversion Constants to Predict Body Fat for YOUNG WOMEN (cont'd.)

| \multicolumn{3}{c|}{Abdomen} | \multicolumn{3}{c|}{Thigh} | \multicolumn{3}{c}{Forearm} |

in	cm	Constant A	in	cm	Constant B	in	cm	Constant C
33.00	83.82	44.12	27.00	68.58	56.17	19.00	48.26	81.90
33.25	84.45	44.45	27.25	69.21	56.69	19.25	48.89	82.98
33.50	85.09	44.78	27.50	69.85	57.21	19.50	49.53	84.05
33.75	85.72	45.12	27.75	70.48	57.73	19.75	50.16	85.13
34.00	86.36	45.45	28.00	71.12	58.26	20.00	50.80	86.21
34.25	86.99	45.79	28.25	71.75	58.78			
34.50	87.63	46.12	28.50	72.39	59.30			
34.75	88.26	46.46	28.75	73.02	59.82			
35.00	88.90	46.79	29.00	73.66	60.34			
35.25	89.53	47.12	29.25	74.29	60.86			
35.50	90.17	47.46	29.50	74.93	61.38			
35.75	90.80	47.79	29.75	75.56	61.90			
36.00	91.44	48.13	30.00	76.20	62.42			
36.25	92.07	48.46	30.25	76.83	62.94			
36.50	92.71	48.80	30.50	77.47	63.46			
36.75	93.34	49.13	30.75	78.10	63.98			
37.00	93.98	49.46	31.00	78.74	64.50			
37.25	94.61	49.80	31.25	79.37	65.02			
37.50	95.25	50.13	31.50	80.01	65.54			
37.75	95.88	50.47	31.75	80.64	66.06			
38.00	96.52	50.80	32.00	81.28	66.58			
38.25	97.15	51.13	32.25	81.91	67.10			
38.50	97.79	51.47	32.50	82.55	67.62			
38.75	98.42	51.80	32.75	83.18	68.14			
39.00	99.06	52.14	33.00	83.82	68.66			
39.25	99.69	52.47	33.25	84.45	69.18			
39.50	100.33	52.81	33.50	85.09	69.70			
39.75	100.96	53.14	33.75	85.72	70.22			
40.00	101.60	53.47	34.00	86.36	70.74			

Young Women: Percent fat = Constant A + Constant B - Constant C - 19.6

Conversion Constants to Predict Body Fat for OLDER WOMEN

\multicolumn{3}{c	}{Abdomen}	\multicolumn{3}{c	}{Thigh}	\multicolumn{3}{c}{Calf}
in	cm	Constant A	in	cm	Constant B	in	cm	Constant C
25.00	63.50	29.69	14.00	35.56	17.31	10.00	25.40	14.46
25.25	64.13	29.98	14.25	36.19	17.62	10.25	26.03	14.82
25.50	64.77	30.28	14.50	36.83	17.93	10.50	26.67	15.18
25.75	65.40	30.58	14.75	37.46	18.24	10.75	27.30	15.54
26.00	66.04	30.87	15.00	38.10	18.55	11.00	27.94	15.91
26.25	66.67	31.17	15.25	38.73	18.86	11.25	28.57	16.27
26.50	67.31	31.47	15.50	39.37	19.17	11.50	29.21	16.63
26.75	67.94	31.76	15.75	40.00	19.47	11.75	29.84	16.99
27.00	68.58	32.06	16.00	40.64	19.78	12.00	30.48	17.35
27.25	69.21	32.36	16.25	41.27	20.09	12.25	31.11	17.71
27.50	69.85	32.65	16.50	41.91	20.40	12.50	31.75	18.08
27.75	70.48	32.95	16.75	42.54	20.71	12.75	32.38	18.44
28.00	71.12	33.25	17.00	43.18	21.02	13.00	33.02	18.80
28.25	71.75	33.55	17.25	43.81	21.33	13.25	33.65	19.16
28.50	72.39	33.84	17.50	44.45	21.64	13.50	34.29	19.52
28.75	73.02	34.14	17.75	45.08	21.95	13.75	34.92	19.88
29.00	73.66	34.44	18.00	45.72	22.26	14.00	35.56	20.24
29.25	74.29	34.73	18.25	46.35	22.57	14.25	36.19	20.61
29.50	74.93	35.03	18.50	46.99	22.87	14.50	36.83	20.97
29.75	75.56	35.33	18.75	47.62	23.18	14.75	37.46	21.33
30.00	76.20	35.62	19.00	48.26	23.49	15.00	38.10	21.69
30.25	76.83	35.92	19.25	48.89	23.80	15.25	38.73	22.05
30.50	77.47	36.22	19.50	49.53	24.11	15.50	39.37	22.41
30.75	78.10	36.51	19.75	50.16	24.42	15.75	40.00	22.77
31.00	78.74	36.81	20.00	50.80	24.73	16.00	40.64	23.14
31.25	79.37	37.11	20.25	51.43	25.04	16.25	41.27	23.50
31.50	80.01	37.40	20.50	52.07	25.35	16.50	41.91	23.86
31.75	80.64	37.70	20.75	52.70	25.66	16.75	42.54	24.22
32.00	81.28	38.00	21.00	53.34	25.97	17.00	43.18	24.58
32.25	81.91	38.30	21.25	53.97	26.28	17.25	43.81	24.94
32.50	82.55	38.59	21.50	54.61	26.58	17.50	44.45	25.31
32.75	83.18	38.89	21.75	55.24	26.89	17.75	45.08	25.67
33.00	83.82	39.19	22.00	55.88	27.20	18.00	45.72	26.03
33.25	84.45	39.48	22.25	56.51	27.51	18.25	46.35	26.39
33.50	85.09	39.78	22.50	57.15	27.82	18.50	46.99	26.75
33.75	85.72	40.08	22.75	57.78	28.13	18.75	47.62	27.11
34.00	86.36	40.37	23.00	58.42	28.44	19.00	48.26	27.47
34.25	86.99	40.67	23.25	59.05	28.75	19.25	48.89	27.84
34.50	87.63	40.97	23.50	59.69	29.06	19.50	49.53	28.20
34.75	88.26	41.26	23.75	60.32	29.37	19.75	50.16	28.56
35.00	88.90	41.56	24.00	60.96	29.68	20.00	50.80	28.92
35.25	89.53	41.86	24.25	61.59	29.98	20.25	51.43	29.28
35.50	90.17	42.15	24.50	62.23	30.29	20.50	52.07	29.64
35.75	90.80	42.45	24.75	62.86	30.60	20.75	52.70	30.00
36.00	91.44	42.75	25.00	63.50	30.91	21.00	53.34	30.37
36.25	92.07	43.05	25.25	64.13	31.22	21.25	53.97	30.73
36.50	92.71	43.34	25.50	64.77	31.53	21.50	54.61	31.09
36.75	93.34	43.64	25.75	65.40	31.84	21.75	55.24	31.45
37.00	93.98	43.94	26.00	66.04	32.15	22.00	55.88	31.81
37.25	94.61	44.23	26.25	66.67	32.46	22.25	56.51	32.17
37.50	95.25	44.53	26.50	67.31	32.77	22.50	57.15	32.54
37.75	95.88	44.83	26.75	67.94	33.08	22.75	57.78	32.90

Section Two

Conversion Constants to Predict Body Fat for OLDER WOMEN (cont'd.)

Abdomen			Thigh			Calf		
in	cm	Constant A	in	cm	Constant B	in	cm	Constant C
38.00	96.52	45.12	27.00	68.58	33.38	23.00	58.42	33.26
38.25	97.15	45.42	27.25	69.21	33.69	23.25	59.05	33.62
38.50	97.79	45.72	27.50	69.85	34.00	23.50	59.69	33.98
38.75	98.43	46.01	27.75	70.48	34.31	23.75	60.32	34.34
39.00	99.06	46.31	28.00	71.12	34.62	24.00	60.96	34.70
39.25	99.69	46.61	28.25	71.75	34.93	24.25	61.59	35.07
39.50	100.33	46.90	28.50	72.39	35.24	24.50	62.23	35.43
39.75	100.96	47.20	28.75	73.02	35.55	24.75	62.86	35.79
40.00	101.60	47.50	29.00	73.66	35.86	25.00	63.50	36.15
40.25	101.24	47.79	29.25	74.29	36.17			
40.50	102.87	48.09	29.50	74.93	36.48			
40.75	103.51	48.39	29.75	75.56	36.79			
41.00	104.14	48.69	30.00	76.20	37.09			
41.25	104.78	48.98	30.25	76.83	37.40			
41.50	105.41	49.28	30.50	77.47	37.71			
41.75	106.05	49.58	30.75	78.10	38.02			
42.00	106.68	49.87	31.00	78.74	38.33			
42.25	107.32	50.17	31.25	79.37	38.64			
42.50	107.95	50.47	31.50	80.01	38.95			
42.75	108.59	50.76	31.75	80.64	39.26			
43.00	109.22	51.06	32.00	81.28	39.57			
43.25	109.86	51.36	32.25	81.91	39.88			
43.50	110.49	51.65	32.50	82.55	40.19			
43.75	111.13	51.95	32.75	83.18	40.49			
44.00	111.76	52.25	33.00	83.82	40.80			
44.25	112.40	52.54	33.25	84.45	41.11			
44.50	113.03	52.84	33.50	85.09	41.42			
44.75	113.67	53.14	33.75	85.72	41.73			
45.00	114.30	53.44	34.00	86.36	42.04			

Older Women: Percent fat = Constant A + Constant B - Constant C - 18.4

Handwritten calculations:

~~11.76~~ + 16.7.31 - 20.24
52.25 + 32.77 - 20.24 - 18.4
85.02 - 20.24 - 18.4
64.78 - 18.4
46.38
8.0809

The Scale Companion

One More Example Before You Start:

The following example shows how to calculate percent body fat, fat weight, and lean body weight for Jim, a hypothetical 21-year-old male who weighs 174 pounds.

Step 1. Measure
Take the girth measurements according to instructions on page 36 and 37. For a 21 year-old male, measurements are taken at the right upper arm, abdomen, and right forearm. The girths are measured twice, and the average recorded to the nearest 0.6 cm (1/4 inch).

<u>Jim's Measurements</u>
Upper arm = 11.5 inches (in.) (29.2 cm.)
Abdomen = 31.0 in. (78.7 cm.)
Right forearm = 10.75 in. (27.3 cm.)

Step 2. Determine the Constants
The table for young men contains the constants A, B, and C corresponding to the three girth measurements from Step 1 for young males.

Constant A, corresponding to 11.5 in. (29.2 cm.) = 42.56
Constant B, corresponding to 31.0 in. (78.7 cm.) = 40.68
Constant C, corresponding to 10.75 in. (27.3 cm.) = 58.37

Step 3. Compute Percent Body Fat
Compute percent body fat by substituting the appropriate constants from Step 2 in the formula shown at the bottom of the table for young males.

% fat = Constant A (upper arm) + Constant B (abdomen)
              − Constant C (right forearm) − 10.2
       = 42.56 + 40.68 − 58.37 − 10.2
       = 83.24 − 58.37 − 10.2
       = 24.87 − 10.2
       = 14.7%

Jim's body fat percentage is 14.7%.

Section Three - Now It's Your Turn

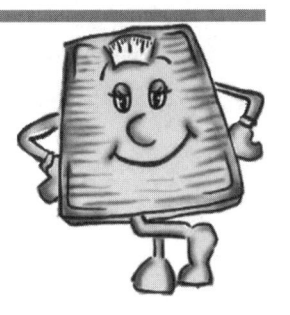

Getting Ready

First, assemble your calculator, tape measure, paper and pencil. Although there is space in this book for you to record your results and make your calculations, you may want to first write them on a separate piece of paper, then transfer the information to this book. Then you won't have to flip your worksheet back and forth between the tables for your age and gender. This book can be a useful ledger to track the changes you make as you exercise, train for strength, and eat more healthfully. If your arm measurement gets smaller you will know you are losing fat in your arm. If your abdomen measurement gets smaller you will know you are losing fat in your mid-section. These decreases mean you are losing fat throughout your body.

The Scale Companion

Step One: Gathering The Data

First, write down your current goal weight. Just for fun, we are going to call it your "fantasy weight."

My fantasy (current goal) weight is: 135 lbs.

After your assessment, you will need to know your scale weight.

My weight today is: 160

Next, go to page 38 and thumb through the charts to determine in which of the four categories you belong. Circle the category appropriate for your statistics:

My age is: 32

I belong in Category: Older Man   (Older Woman)
                         Younger Man   Younger Woman

Next, go to page 36 and, based on your category, record which of the three sites you will measure.

The three sites I will measure:
Abd   thigh   Calf

The bottom of your chart also provides the appropriate formula to use after you have taken your measurements.

Write yours here: Constant A + Constant B - Constant C -18

Section Three

Following the instructions on page 36 and 37, take your measurements and record them below. Take the measurement at least twice (preferably in centimeters), average the two numbers and record the result.

My measurements are:

Site one is: __92 - abd__

    My first measurement is: __92__

    My second measurement is: __62__

    The average of these two measurements is: __92__ (1)

Site two is: __(r) calf__

    My first measurement is: __61__

    My second measurement is: __62__

    The average of these two measurements is: __61.5__ (2)

Site three is: __(r) calf__

    My first measurement is: __35__

    My second measurement is: __35__

    The average of these two measurements is: __35__ (3)

The Scale Companion

Now you are ready to return to the chart appropriate for your age and gender category, and convert these measurements into constants.

Measurement one: _abd_ (1) Constant A is: _92_

Measurement two: _thigh_ (2) Constant B is: _61_

Measurement three: _calf_ (3) Constant C is: _35_

On the bottom of page 48 you wrote down the calculation necessary to convert these constants to percent body fat.

Rewrite the formula and do the math here:

$$A + B - C - 18.4$$

73.03 -   153 - 35 - 18.4

118 - 18.4

43.05 (A)   29.98 (B)

20.24 (C)   5.12 — 52.79

My percent body fat is: _34.4_

As you read earlier, experts generally agree that 20-30% fat is a healthy body fat range for women and 10-20% fat is a healthy body fat range for men. If your body fat percentage fell within these goals, give yourself a pat on the back. You can still complete the calculations that will assure your goal weight is appropriate. If your result fell outside these average ranges, don't panic. This assessment is a benchmark you can use to calculate a realistic weight.

Section Three

Step Two: Using The Data

Now you will want to compute your pounds of fat and pounds of lean mass. The latter number will provide you with the information necessary to compute a realistic goal weight.

First, compute your pounds of fat. Multiply your current weight by your percent body fat. To get an accurate result, be sure to convert your percent body fat to a decimal. This is accomplished by putting a decimal in front of the body fat percentage result. (For example, if you are a woman whose body fat percentage is 33%, you would multiply your current weight by 0.33.)

Now calculate your pounds of fat:

Actual weight X body fat percent = pounds of fat.

    160 X .34   54.4

The next calculation reveals the weight of your fat-free or lean mass. (For this purpose we are going to use these terms interchangeably.) The higher this number is, the better. To find your pounds of fat-free mass, subtract your pounds of fat from your current weight.

Now calculate your pounds of fat-free mass:

Current weight − pounds of fat = pounds of fat-free mass.

    160 − 54.4 =   105.6

Step Three: Calculating Your Ideal Weight

Now you're ready to calculate your ideal weight.

First, choose a desired body fat goal. (See the bottom of page 21 for a reminder of optimum goals for men and women.) Next, subtract that number from 100 to learn what percentage of your weight, at goal, will be lean mass. Convert that number to a decimal. To calculate your realistic goal weight, divide this number into your current lean mass.

100 - desired body fat % = % of desired lean body mass.

Convert that number to a decimal and divide it into your current lean mass to learn you ideal weight.

Current lean mass ÷ percentage of desired lean body mass (expressed as a decimal) = realistic goal weight.

For example: If a female client with a current weight of 150 pounds has a current body fat percentage of 30%, she has 45 pounds of fat and 105 pounds of lean mass. If she chooses a body fat goal of 25% she subtracts that number from 100% to learn her % of lean mass at goal. (100% - 25% = 75%) That percentage is converted to a decimal and divided into her current lean mass to calculate her ideal weight.

105 ÷ .75 = 140 pounds
140 pounds is her realistic weight.

Now do your calculations:

100 - __25__ = __.75__
     (your desired body fat)   (your desired lean mass)

__105.6__ ÷ __.75__ = _____
(your current lean mass) (your desired lean mass   (your ideal weight)
                           expressed as decimal)

My ideal goal weight is: __140__.

Section Three

Surprising Results!

In our experience, people who have a large lean mass (because they are active or overweight or genetically predisposed to be more muscular) are surprised to discover that their realistic goal weight is much higher than the goal weight they wrote down on page 48. That original goal weight was unreasonable.

Now that you have calculated a realistic goal weight, you can calculate (excuse the pun) your bottom line. How many pounds of fat do you need to lose to reach that realistic weight? To find out, subtract your realistic goal weight from your current weight.

Calculate the pounds of fat you need to lose here:
Current weight − realistic goal weight = pounds of fat to lose.

I have __20__ pounds of fat to lose to reach my realistic goal weight.

You don't need to look at charts any more. Your goal weight is no longer arbitrary- it is based on who you are today and what you can do to be as healthy as possible.

A Fantasy Calculation

If you started this process with an unrealistic goal weight, you might enjoy knowing how low your body fat would have to be to reach that goal. We call this a "fantasy" body fat goal. Divide your current lean by your fantasy weight, then subtract the answer from 100.

To illustrate this, let's look again at Marie's numbers. Marie wanted to weigh 125 pounds (her fantasy weight). Her assessment of 35% fat showed a lean mass of 97.5 pounds.

Current lean ÷ original goal weight = fantasy body fat goal.

97.5 ÷ 125 = 0.78.

100 – 78 = 22%.

In order to satisfy Marie's 125 pound fantasy weight, she would have to decrease her body fat percentage from her current 35% to 22%. The five-pound difference between Marie's ideal weight and her fantasy weight yielded a 3% difference in body fat.

Your calculation here:

Remember, your ideal weight is no longer based on height/weight charts, what you weighed when you were younger or any other criteria! It is based solely on *how much lean mass you have today.*

Section Four: Smart Resources

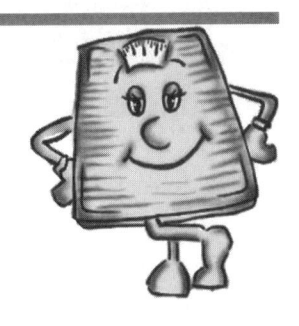

The Rest Of YOUR Story

If you opened this book because you were unhappy with your current weight we hope *THE SCALE COMPANION* has given you the information you need to support a change in your attitude in regard to what your weight should be. If you are already at a satisfactory goal weight, *THE SCALE COMPANION* can be used to help you maintain that goal.

If your goal is weight management, remember exercise plays a valuable role in successful long term weight management. It is not the purpose of this book to provide exercise or dietary guidelines. Seek professional guidance to help you design an exercise program that specifically meets your needs. Co-author of this booklet, Ronda Gates, has also authored **SMART EATING**. It provides excellent guidelines for choosing wisely and living lean. You can find it at any bookstore or order an autographed copy by using the toll free number on page 58 of our resource section.

If you want professional day-to-day, one-on-one, weight management coaching contact a registered dietitian or consider Ronda's web coaching services.

Beyond that, we offer you our encouragement and support. We believe in a lifelong, lowfat lifestyle "on the go." We hope we have helped you get off to a good start!

Other Books Published by Authors:

College Texts

Check out our college textbooks (1-800-638-0672; visit the publisher on the Internet. http://www.wwilkins.com).

McArdle, W. D., Katch, F. I. and Katch, V. L. *Exercise Physiology: Food, Energy, and Human Performance.* Fourth Edition. Williams & Wilkins, Baltimore, 1996. 849 pages.

Katch, F. I. and W. D. McArdle. *Introduction to Nutrition, Exercise, and Health.* Fourth Edition. (formerly Nutrition, Weight Control, and Exercise) Lea & Febiger, Philadelphia, 1993. 587 pages.

McArdle, W. D., Katch, F. I. and Katch, V. L. *Essentials of Exercise Physiology.* Williams & Wilkins, Baltimore, 1994. 563 pages.

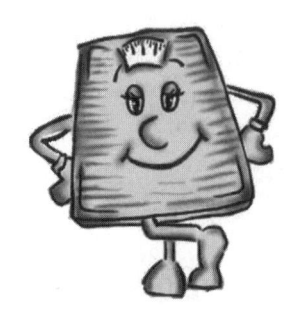

Section Four

Additional Reading

We have also written other books. Some are useful for students pursuing fitness as a career. Some are useful for everybody. They include:

Katch, F. I., Katch, V.L. and W.D. McArdle. *Career Planning, Resume Writing, and Job Placement.* Fitness Technologies Press. Ann Arbor, MI, 1996. 54 pages. $11.95.

Katch, V. L., Katch, F. I. and W. D. McArdle. *Directory of Graduate Programs. Exercise Science, Physical Therapy, Physician Assistant, and Occupational Therapy.* Fitness Technologies Press. Ann Arbor, MI, 1996. 150 pages. $18.95.

Katch, V. L., Katch, F. I. and W. D. McArdle. *Crosswords for Exercise Physiology.* Fitness Technologies Press. Ann Arbor, MI, 1996. 145 pages. $9.95.

To order the 3 books above direct: Fitness Technologies Press. 1132 Lincoln Avenue. Ann Arbor, MI 48104. Price includes shipping 4th class mail and handling. Outside North America, add $5. Checks and money orders in US currency only. No Credit Cards. (For 1st class: USA add $4.00 first item, $1.25 each additional item; outside North America add $12.00 first item, $2.00 each additional item).

Katch, V. L., Katch, F. I. and W. D. McArdle. *Calorie Expenditure Charts.* Fitness Technologies Press. Ann Arbor, MI, 1996. Order from Fitness Technologies Press or LIFESTYLES by Ronda Gates, 1-800-863-6000. $11.95

Bailey, Covert and Gates, Ronda. *Smart Eating.* Houghton Mifflin. Boston, MA, 1996. 256 pages. Order from LIFESTYLES by Ronda Gates, 1-800-863-6000. $9.95

Gates, Ronda. *Nutrition Nuggets/Changes–The Rest of the Story.* LIFESTYLES 4-Heart Press. Lake Oswego, OR, 1993. 256 pages. Order from LIFESTYLES by Ronda Gates, 1-800-863-6000. $8.00

Gates, Ronda and Parker, Valerie. *The Lowfat Lifestyle*. LIFESTYLES 4-Heart Press. Lake Oswego, OR, 1986, 256 pages. Order from LIFESTYLES by Ronda Gates, 1-800-863-6000.

Mailing Addresses:

Ronda Gates, P. O. Box 974, Lake Oswego, OR 97034

Frank Katch, Department of Exercise Science, University of Massachusetts, Amherst, MA 01003

Victor Katch, Department of Kinesiology, University of Michigan, Ann Arbor, MI 48104

E-mail Addresses:

Ronda Gates: rondagates@aol.com

Frank Katch: fkatch@excsci.umass.edu

Victor Katch: vkass@umich.edu

Our World Wide Web Sites:

Ronda Gates: http://www.rondagates.com

Speaking Services And Program Development:

To reach any of us for information on our speaking services or other programs and products we have developed contact: LIFESTYLES by Ronda Gates, P. O. Box 974, Lake Oswego, OR 97034; Phone: 503-697-7572; or call toll free 1-800-863-6000

Ronda Gates

Currently employed: Entrepreneur owner of LIFESTYLES by Ronda Gates, which develops and delivers health promotion programs and products to support change.

Other professional kudos: Certified Lifestyle Counselor with emphasis in weight control and stress management, Certified by American College of Sports Medicine as a Fitness Leader, Elected Fellow Association of Worksite Health Promotion, Master Trainer and Sr. Development Team member of Reebok University, qualified provider of Myers Briggs Type Indicator, published author of ***Lowfat Lifestyle, Nutrition Nuggets and Smart Eating***

What she enjoys: Motivational speaking, teaching fitness classes, the challenge of PacNW gardening, E-mail

Where you are sure to find her smiling: MacWorld conventions, bragging about her favorite musicians (her children, Rebecca and Caleb), on a tennis court, traveling with friends, at the theater

Where she lives: Lake Oswego, OR

Favorite foods: Caesar Salad, pizza, milk chocolate brownies

Pet peeve: People who make promises they won't keep, people who tell me what I'm thinking or feeling.

Frank Katch

Currently employed: Professor of Exercise Science at the University of Massachusetts at Amherst

Other kudos: Elected to the American Academy of Kinesiology, Fellow of the American College of Sports Medicine, reviewer for numerous scientific journals, co-author of the classic college text, ***Nutrition, Weight Control, and Exercise*** (4th edition), ***Exercise Physiology, Energy, Nutrition, and Human Performance*** (4th edition), and forthcoming book, ***Exercise and Sports Nutrition.***

What he enjoys: Writing, biking, jogging trails in cities he visits, surfing the net on his Apple Power Mac, sports and nature photography, trying to figure out a way to win the lottery for early retirement.

Where you can be sure to find him smiling: MacWorld conventions, vacationing in Carmel, CA, walks with his wife Kerry, and enjoying his 3 children (David, Kevin, and Ellen)

Where he lives: Amherst, MA

Favorite food: Homemade meatloaf smothered in ketchup and onions, enchiladas, and fancy-named ice cream (any kind).

Pet peeve: Listening to people complain about gaining weight without wanting to exercise!

Victor Katch

Currently employed: Professor of Kinesiology, Associate Professor of Pediatric Cardiology, University of Michigan, Ann Arbor, Michigan. Director Behnke Body Composition Laboratory and Advanced Fitness Training Center.

Other professional kudos: Elected to American Academy of Kinesiology, Reviewer for numerous scientific journals, co-authors of classic college text; ***Exercise Physiology: Energy, Nutrition, and Human Performance*** (4th Edition), forthcoming text, ***Exercise and Sports Nutrition***, author of ***Allied Health Program Directory***, and ***Calorie Expenditure Charts for Physical Activity: The complete resource of calories burned during household, occupational, and sport and physical fitness activities.*** Received outstanding teacher awards from School of Kinesiology, 1995.

What he enjoys: Walking and jogging on beach, reading magazines, playing with his 2 year old son, Jesse, joking and shopping with his daughters, Erika and Leslie, listening to talk radio.

Where you are sure to find him smiling: Spending time with wife Heather; messing with electronic gadgets

Where he lives: Ann Arbor, Michigan, the best college town in America.

Favorite foods: French toast, kiwi, passion fruit

Pet peeve: Lights not turned out when people leave the room, people who leave "things" on my desk.

NOTES: